Medical Math

Gaining Competency with Medical Math

Medical Math: Gaining Competency with Medical Math

ISBN: 978-0-9897596-2-5

Published by Hidden Valley Publishing L.L.C.
Idaho, U.S.A.
http://hiddenvalleypublishing.com

Acknowledgements

First of all, I would like to thank my incredible medical math professor, Mr. William S. Blair. He made math applicable to me and impressed upon me its importance- so much so that I wanted to share it with others through this quick resource guide.

I cannot express enough thanks to my wife for her love, support and encouragement. She not only put up with me working long hours late into the night but she also provided insight about how to better explain some of the mathematical problems.

Additionally, I want to thank my sister Rachel Sanchez, RN for reviewing each of the questions in the book and providing feedback on improving the questions to help students better understand the type of questions they will face when working in the medical field.

Table of Contents

Introduction

On the first day of my medical math class, the professor began class by reading the headlines of various articles that read something like this: “Mother of 4 dies due to nurse administering lethal dose”, “5-year old boy dies due to overdose” or “Man suffers cardiac arrest due to wrong drug administered”.

We learned that medical errors in hospitals kill more Americans every year than AIDS, breast cancer and auto accidents combined.

Some first day huh?

I decided that I would study and learn all there was to know about reading drug orders, measuring dose amounts and administering the drugs according to the doctors’ orders. Patients and family members place a lot of trust in our skills and training. This was not a class to take lightly.

Studies have shown that students tend to only remember roughly 20% of what they learned in class! That’s not a very good percentage for those training to be in healthcare where a mistake could be lethal.

This book is a basic guidebook for those preparing for a medical math class, currently enrolled in one, or a handy guide for those who have already taken it but would like a quick place to brush up on those skills.

Notes/Calculations

Metric System

Health care providers use the metric system when ordering and measuring drugs for patients. The **metric system** is an international standard of measurement based on decimals. It is used to measure weight (mcg, mg, g, kg), volume (ml, L), and length (mm, cm, m). See chart below. It is vital that you have the Metric System memorized so that you can perform Dimensional Analysis.

Metric System Prefixes

Prefix	Fraction form	Decimal	Exponent	Example	Meaning
mc (micro-)	$\frac{1}{1,000,000}$	0.000001	10^{-6}	mcg	One millionth of a gram
m (milli-)	$\frac{1}{1,000}$	0.001	10^{-3}	mL	One thousandth of a liter
c (centi-)	$\frac{1}{100}$	0.01	10^{-2}	cm	One hundredth of a meter
d (deci-)	$\frac{1}{10}$	0.1	10^{-1}	dL	One tenth of a liter
k (kilo-)	1000	1000	10^{3}	kg	One thousand grams

Metric System conversion factors

Weight	Volume	Length
1000mcg = 1mg	1000mL = 1L	1000mm = 1m
1000mg = 1g	-	100cm = 1m
1000g = 1kg	-	10mm = 1cm

Pound to kg conversion: 1 kg = 2.2 lbs

cc = Cubic cm

1cc = 1mL

Notes/Calculations

When learning the metric system units it helps to compare those smaller units of measurements to the standard units that most Americans use on a daily basis. In the chart below, we compare the Metric Systems Volume, expressed in millimeters or mL to the standard household units.

	Household						
	Teaspoon	*Tablespoon*	*Ounce*	*Cup*	*Pint*	*Quarts*	*Gallon*
Metric							
5mL	1tsp						
15mL	3tsp	1tbs					
30mL		2tbs	1oz				
240mL			8oz	1cup			
500mL				2cups	1pint		
1,000mL					2pints	1quart	
4,000mL						4quarts	1gal

It is important to note that the mL used in the chart above doesn't correlate exactly with the Household units but rather an even rounded number that is often used when preforming medical math problems. For example; there are 236.588mL in 1 US cup and 473.176mL in two US cups. We will round the numbers to 240mL and 500mL respectively.

Understanding the chart

Only values in the vertical columns correlate to each other. For example; 30mL is equivalent to 2tbs which is also the same as 1oz. Additionally, 240mL is the same as saying 8oz or 1 cup.

Let's say we wanted to know how many mL are in 2.5quarts. We know that there are 1,000 mL in 1quart so we can double that to get 2 quarts or 2,000mL and then divide one quart in half (1,000 / 2 = 500), now we add the 500 to the 2,000 and we have 2,500mL or 2.5quarts.

Temperature Conversion

Celsius to Fahrenheit – (Add 40, multiply by 1.8 then subtract 40)
Fahrenheit to Celsius – (Add 40, divide by 1.8, then subtract 40)
Example: *47 degrees Celsius to Fahrenheit* (47 + 40 x 1.8 – 40 = **116.6 F.**)

Notes/Calculations

Here are some sample questions to help you practice memorizing the conversion charts.

1- Write the name for the prefix "m". _______

2- Write what Kg means. ________

3- Write the abbreviation for the prefix that means 1,000 ._______

4- Write the abbreviation for the prefix that means 1/1,000.________

5- Write the name for the base unit of weight, or mass.________

6- Write the abbreviation for the base unit of volume.________

7- Write the meaning for the base unit 1/10._______

8- Write the meaning for the base unit 1/1,000,000.__________

Correct Metric Abbreviations

Circle the correct answer in the questions below. If you need help you can refer back to page 3.

milliliters - m - mg - mL - mml	**microgram** - mG - mcg - mL - Mg	**grams** - gm - g - mcg - mml
milligrams - m - mgm - mL - mg	**liters** - l - lT - L - lt	**Kilogram** - KG - lbs - kgs - Kg

Notes/Calculations

Setting up your DA equation

In the medical field we use a mathematical process called **Dimensional Analysis**(DA). There are a few simple guidelines to be aware of when setting up your problems. They consist of the following:

Steps	**Process**
1	Identify the desired units for the answer
2	Identify your "on-hand" units
3	Identify the needed conversion factors
4	Determine the correct structure for the problem
5	Estimate the answer
6	Perform the necessary mathematics
7	Evaluate the answer and compare to your estimated answer

Example

100mg is equal to how many g?

$$g \quad \frac{100mg}{} \;\Big|\; \frac{1g}{1000mg} = \boxed{0.1g}$$

Let's take a look at the example used above as we do each of the 7 steps of the DA equation.

Step1: Identify the desired units for the answer.

In the example shown above, we need to know how many g is equivalent to 100mg? First, write down the desired units as g.

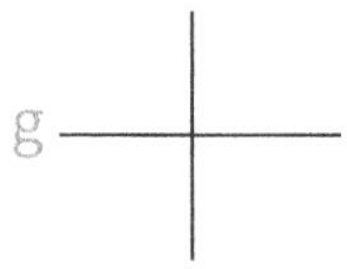

Step2: Identify your "on-hand" units.

The units we have on hand in this example are 100mg.

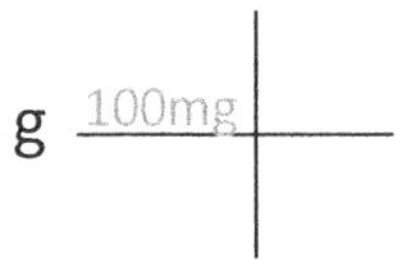

Notes/Calculations

Step3: Identify the needed conversion factors.

Here is where your hard work in memorizing the chart on page 3 pays off. We know that there are 1000mg in 1g.

g	100mg	

1000mg = 1g

Step4: Determine the correct structure for the problem.

If you remember way back to grade school math, in order to cross cancel units, the units cannot be on the same side of the division as each other. In other words, if you have mg on the top (*numerator*) then the other unit must be on the bottom (*denominator*).

***See the discussion note on page 13 about setting up your conversion factors.*

g	100mg (mg cancelled)	1g
		1000mg

Step5: Estimate the answer.

By estimating the answer, you will be able to catch yourself from making any mathematical errors. For example, in our problem we used a conversion factor of 1g = 1000mg. We know that the answer should come out to be around 0.1 and not 1.0 because 1g is 1000x bigger than a mg.

Notes/Calculations

DA Equation Continued (2nd part)

Step6: Preform the necessary mathematics.

Working from left to right, cancel units (*Numerator mg – Denominator mg*) until you are left with just your desired units of g. Next multiply the numerator across (100 x 1 = 100). Then do the same with the denominator (1 x 1000 = 1000). Next, divide the new numerator by the denominator (100 / 1000 = 0.1). Finally, grams is all that is left so you carry it to your answer. (0.1g).

$$g \quad \frac{100\,\cancel{mg}}{} \Big| \frac{1g}{1000\,\cancel{mg}} = 0.1g$$

Step7: Evaluate the answer and compare to your estimated answer from step5.

We estimated that the final answer would be around 0.1g and after doing our DA analysis we have concluded that our answer does match our estimated answer from step 5.

Discussion:

It is important to note that when structuring your equation in <u>step 4</u> you place the conversion factor in the correct order. In our example above, we wanted to know how many **g** are equivalent to **100mg**. As such we used the conversion of 1g = 1000mg. We placed the 1g in the numerator and the 1000mg in the denominator because we are seeking an answer in **g**.

Notes/Calculations

In this section we want to focus on selecting the correct setup for our DA equations. In each problem circle the correct Conversion Factor setup for the desired units to the problem.

> The trick here lies within the numerator/dominator cancelation rule that we discussed earlier. In order for us to "cancel out" the unit we start with, it needs to be diagonal from it in the conversion factor. If we are starting with the units in feet for example in number 1 and converting it to inches, then we are starting with ft/1 (just like any number over one is itself we can assume that rule with units). With this rule, then every conversion factor should be the (desired unit/original unit).

1- How many inches are in a foot?

Desired Units	Conversion Factors
in	$\frac{1\text{ft}}{12\text{in}}$ OR $\frac{12\text{in}}{1\text{ft}}$

2- How many kilometers are in 6 miles?

Desired Units	Conversion Factors
km	$\frac{0.6\text{mile}}{1\text{km}}$ OR $\frac{1\text{km}}{0.6\text{mile}}$

3- How many ounces are in 15 pounds?

Desired Units	Conversion Factors
oz	$\frac{1\text{lbs}}{16\text{oz}}$ OR $\frac{16\text{oz}}{1\text{lbs}}$

Notes/Calculations

You should be able to fill out this chart by *memory*.

1tsp	ml
1tbs	tsp
3oz	ml
1g	mcg
1in	cm
1m	cm

In the following table, fill in the required amounts – **SHOW ALL WORK**

0.7g	mg	
100mg	g	
4m	cm	
400cm	m	
12in	cm	
25mm	cm	

Notes/Calculations

Sometimes we need to use more than one set of conversion factors to arrive at our desired units. This is easy to do if you have the correct set of factors that share units. In this section we are going to take a look at some sample questions and determine how many conversion factors we will need.

1- How many inches are in a yard?

# of Conversion Factors	Possible Conversion Factors	Show Work
	12in = 1ft 1in = 2.54cm 3ft = 1yd 39in = 1m 1in = 25.4mm 1yd = 91.4cm 1L = 1000mL 1qt = 1L 4qt = 1gal	

2- How many mL are in a gal?

# of Conversion Factors	Possible Conversion Factors	Show Work
	12in = 1ft 1in = 2.54cm 3ft = 1yd 39in = 1m 1in = 25.4mm 1yd = 91.4cm 1L = 1000mL 1qt = 1L 4qt = 1gal	

3- How many cm are in 3yd?

# of Conversion Factors	Possible Conversion Factors	Show Work
	12in = 1ft 1in = 2.54cm 3ft = 1yd 39in = 1m 1in = 25.4mm 1yd = 91.4cm 1L = 1000mL 1qt = 1L 4qt = 1gal	

4- How many cm are in 1ft?

# of Conversion Factors	Possible Conversion Factors	Show Work
	12in = 1ft 1in = 2.54cm 3ft = 1yd 39in = 1m 1in = 25.4mm 1yd = 91.4cm 1L = 1000mL 1qt = 1L 4qt = 1gal	

Notes/Calculations

How many tbs are in 8oz?	**Show Work** tbs = $\frac{2\,tbs}{1\,oz} \times \frac{8\,oz}{}$ = 2 x 8 = 16tbs
How many tsp are in 1pint?	**Show Work**
How many mcg are in 350mg?	**Show Work**
270mcg is equivalent to how many g?	**Show Work**
274mL is equivalent to how many L?	**Show Work**
How many pounds are in 75kg?	**Show Work**
75mm is equivalent to how many cm?	**Show Work**

Notes/Calculations

How many minutes are in 0.3hr?	Show Work $\text{min} = \frac{0.3\ \text{hr}}{} \Big\vert \frac{60\ \text{min}}{1\ \text{hr}}$ = .3 x 60 = 18 min
How many m are in 30yd?	Show Work
How many mm are in 1in?	Show Work
How many cups are in 3.5qt?	Show Work
How many inches are in 65yd?	Show Work
How many kg are in 15 lbs?	Show Work
How many seconds are in 3.5min?	Show Work

Notes/Calculations

Milligram-to-Gram

Milligram	*Gram*
70	0.07g
1000	
3000	
400	
350	

EXAMPLE

$$g \quad \frac{70\ mg}{\ } \Big| \frac{1g}{1000mg} = \mathbf{0.07g}$$

Gram-to-Milligram

Gram	*Milligram*
0.25	250mg
2	
0.8	
0.145	
0.05	

EXAMPLE

$$mg \quad \frac{0.25g}{\ } \Big| \frac{1000mg}{1g} = \mathbf{250mg}$$

Discussion:
When converting milligrams to grams or grams to milligrams you can simply move the decimal three spaces. If you'll notice in the above example, 0.25g is the same as 250mg, we simply moved the decimal to the right 3 spaces because we were multiplying by 1000. Additionally, when we divide by 1000 we would move the decimal to the left 3 spaces.

Notes/Calculations

Let's take a look at some real world problems you may face while working as a nurse! We will only be working with Milligrams-to-Grams.

1- The patient's doctor ordered 1.8g of Drug X. What is the dose in terms of mg?

2- The patient's doctor ordered 0.8g of Drug Y. What is the dose in terms of mg?

3- The patient's doctor ordered 3.6g of Drug Z. What is the dose in terms of mg?

4- The patient's doctor ordered 0.006g of Drug A. What is the dose in terms of mg?

Notes/Calculations

1- The patient's doctor ordered 8,610mg of Drug X. What is the dose in terms of g?

2- The patient's doctor ordered 910mg of Drug X. What is the dose in terms of g?

3- The patient's doctor ordered 25mg of Drug X. What is the dose in terms of g?

4- The patient's doctor ordered 1,801mg of Drug X. What is the dose in terms of g?

Notes/Calculations

1- The patient's doctor ordered 2,800mcg of Drug X. What is the dose in terms of g?

2- The patient's doctor ordered 20,000mcg of Drug X. What is the dose in terms of g?

3- The patient's doctor ordered 5000mcg of Drug X. What is the dose in terms of g?

4- The patient's doctor ordered 23,500mcg of Drug X. What is the dose in terms of g?

Notes/Calculations

1- 0.35L of medication is how many mL?

2- If you drank 34oz of medication, what is the equivalent amount in tbs?

3- The patient's doctor ordered 3.5tbs of Drug X. How many oz is that equal to?

4- The patient's doctor ordered 1.5L of Drug A into the I.V. line. What is the equivalent amount in mL?

Notes/Calculations

cap: (capsule)	Medication covered in a hard or soft gelatin. Capsules come in various sizes. You should never cut or divide capsules into smaller amounts.
tab: (tablet)	Medication combined with powder and formed into tablets.
ung: (ointment)	Oily or cream base medication applied to the skin.
***CD:** (controlled-dose) Sustained Action	A tablet that releases or delays the release of the medication at specified doses and timed intervals.
***DS:** (double-strength)	A tablet or caplet that has double the amount of medication contained within the same size of a standard tablet or caplet.
***LA:** (Long-acting)	Medication that maintains its effects over a long period of time after the initial dosage.
***SR:** (slow-release)	A tablet that is used to maintain *balanced levels* of the drug in the blood for the duration of the medication life.
***XL:** (extra-long-acting)	A tablet that has a longer medication life.
***XR:** (extended-release)	A tablet that has a longer period of releasing time into the bloodstream.

* **Time release terminology** doesn't have an industry standard so it is important that you write out these abbreviations clear and always ask if you are unsure of the term used. Additionally, the time release terms refer to the mechanism used in a tablet, capsule or any other pill to release the medication slower, steadier and/or longer into the bloodstream.

aq: (aqueous)	Medication mixed with a water-based solution.
elix: (elixir)	A sweetened liquid containing alcohol that is used in medication.
emul: (emulsion)	A mixture of two different liquids that are not normally mixed together.
fld: (fluid)	Containing fluid composition.
mixt: (mixture)	Medication consisting of two or more liquid medication.
sol: (solution)	A water based medication.
***susp:** (suspension)	Medication that has solid particles mixed with liquid.
Compound	Medication containing two or more drugs.
Enteric-coated table	A tablet covered with a coating that delays absorption until it reaches the intestines. It is designed to protect the mouth, esophageal, & gastric mucosa.
Scored tablet	Tablet that is scored (cut in the tablet) that it may be split in half.

* **Suspension-** Medication must be thoroughly mixed immediately before it is administered to the patient.

Notes/Calculations

Nonparenteral vs Parenteral

There are two main ways medication can be introduced into the body. **Nonparenteral (**Non-injectable**)** and **Parenteral (**Injectable**).** For the noninjectables there are several different ways the medication can be administered. For example: oral, nasogastric, enteric (Intestinal), rectal, topical, gastric, vaginal, eyes & ears.

Nonparenteral Medication routes

ABBREVIATION or TERMS	ROUTES
Buccal (bucc)	Dissolved in the cheek, not swallowed
SL, subl	Dissolved under the tongue, not swallowed
Ear & Eyes	Left or Right ear/eye (Always write out, Do not abbreviate)
GT	Administered via a Gastrostomy tube
enteric	Administered via a tube directly to the stomach
MDI	Metered dose inhaler
NG (T)	Administered via a Nasogastric tube
Rectal	"Per rectum" (Always write out, Do not abbreviate)
Vag	Administered via the Vagina
NPO	Nothing by mouth
PO	Given by mouth
Top	Administered via topical (applied to the skin)

Parenteral Medication routes

ABBREVIATION or TERMS	ROUTES
IM	Intramuscular; injected into the muscle tissue
ID	Intradermal; injected into the dermal layer
IV	Intravenous; injected into the vein
IVPB	Intravenous piggyback; secondary small bag attached to main IV
epidural	Administered into the epidural space (lower lumbar space)
hypo	Hypodermic; "Under the skin" (Subcutaneous & IM)
subcut	Subcutaneous; injected under the skin
intrathecal	injected into the spinal canal

Notes/Calculations

The time and frequency of medication to be administered is just as important as what type of medication is to be administered and where the medication is to be administered.

Giving the correct medication with the correct amount of medication at the wrong time or frequency can be just as harmful as giving the wrong type of medication.

Below is a chart with the abbreviations and terms of the frequency/time used in the medical field.

Medication Frequency and Time

ABBREVIATION or TERMS	MEANING
$\bar{a}$ or a	Before
$\bar{p}$	After
$\bar{c}$	With
$\bar{s}$	Without
ac	Before meals
pc	After meals
ad lib	Give as desired (fluids and activity only)
bid	Two times a day
tid	Three times a day
qid	Four times a day
prn	As needed
q	Each/every
qh	Every hour
q2h	Every 2 hours
q5h	Every 5 hours
q12h	Every 12 hours
qhs	Every night at bedtime
stat	Give medication immediately (only once)

Notes/Calculations

Fill in the chart below with the appropriate abbreviation or term. If an abbreviation is not recommended, then write out the appropriate term. Some of the terms provided are not real terms, in that case, write "Not a real term" in the answer space provided. Remember, if you are unsure of what the doctor is requesting then ASK for further clarification.

Term	Answer	Term	Answer
IV		Given by Mouth	
$\bar{s}$		IVPB	
rectal		Bid	
GT		Top	
q4h		prn	
diq		Without	
$\bar{a}$		Two times a day	
Ear L		before meals	
ac		Oral	
sub		hypo	
IM		subcut	
ad lib		R eye	
subl		Metered dose inhaler	
With		bucc	
q8h		NG (T)	
Ps		As needed	
Stat		epidural	
ID		SL	
pc		Each, every	
enteric		$\breve{c}$	
tid		Given by Mouth	

Notes/Calculations

The 24-hour clock is also known as military time or international time. The clock always has four digits regardless of the time. The first two digits are designated as the hour and the last two digits are for the minutes. For example: 0200 = 2:00am, 1400 = 2:00pm, or 0235 = 2:35am, and 1435 = 2:35pm.

A few key points to know

- Add 12 hours to the current time in the standard time (1:00PM = 1300 ***12+1**)
- Midnight is 0000 or 2400 depending upon the agency
- AM or PM are not used in military time
- The AM clock is from 2400 hours (Midnight) – 1159 hours (11:59am)
- The PM Clock is from 1200 hours (noon) – 2359 hours (11:59pm)

See the chart below

12-hr clock	**24-hr clock**
Midnight 12:00am	**2400**
1:00 AM	0100
2:00 AM	0200
3:00 AM	0300
4:00 AM	0400
5:00 AM	0500
6:00 AM	0600
7:00 AM	0700
8:00 AM	0800
9:00 AM	0900
10:00 AM	1000
11:00 AM	1100

AM Clock
2400 hours (Midnight) –
1159 hours (11:59am)

12-hr clock	**24-hr clock**
Noon 12:00pm	**1200**
1:00 PM	1300
2:00 PM	1400
3:00 PM	1500
4:00 PM	1600
5:00 PM	1700
6:00 PM	1800
7:00 PM	1900
8:00 PM	2000
9:00 PM	2100
10:00 PM	2200
11:00 PM	2300

PM Clock
1200 hours (noon) –
2359 hours (11:59pm)

Notes/Calculations

ABBREVIATION or TERMS	MEANING
Generic Drug	Official name used for the drug by all companies
NKA	No Known Allergies
NKDA	No Known Drug Allergies
Trade Name	Name assigned to the drug by its manufacture. Usually has ®
Unit Dose	Single Serving of a drug. Ex: 100mg per tablet or 160mg per 5mL
Usual Dose	The recommended dose for the drug. Ex: 1-2 tablets every 4- 6 hours

Circle the best answer:

1- How many times a day is a q6h medication given?

a. 4 c. 12
b. 3 d. 6

2- What is the time in standard time for 0001 and 0333?

a. 12:01/3:33AM
c. 1AM/3:33AM
b. 1AM/ 3:33PM
d. 12:01 /3:33PM

3- Starting at 0001 name the time a drug is administered q3h?

____

4- Write out the doctor's orders in your own words.
"Drug X 500mcg/kg q4h stat"

____

5- What is the correct interpretation of the doctor's orders?
"Morphine 8mg IM stat and q6h"

____

Notes/Calculations

You will be required to understand how to read drug labels ensuring that the patients get the correct amount of the drug they are prescribed by their doctor. Below is an illustration of what a drug label may look like. You will need to know the main parts to correctly read the drug label.

Label	Part
NDC0663-5391-71	
250 Capsules	Total amount of Capsules in bottle
Principen©	Registered Trade Name
Ampicillin	Generic Name
Capsules, USP	Medication form
250mg	Unit Dose amount
CAUTION: Federal law prohibits dispensing without prescription. **Usual Dose**: Adults 1-2 tablets	

Let's say that the doctor's order is:

500mg of Principen @ bid.

How many tablets are you going to give the patient? How many in a day?

The correct answer is 2 tablets now and 2 tablets later.

Fill in the correct information regarding the drug label.

Total amount:____________________

Trade Name:______________________

Generic Name:____________________

Medication Form:_________________

Unit Dose:_______________________

Usual Amount:____________________

NDC0663-5391-71

75mL

Zofran©

Ondansetron hydrochloride

Oral Solution

3mg / 5mL

CAUTION: Federal law prohibits dispensing without prescription.

Usual Dose: Adults 5-10 mL

Notes/Calculations

A patient is prescribed Tegretol to treat his nerve pain. The doctor tells you to give him 510 mg bid. Which container are you going to get the medication from? _________

Container 1

NDC0663-5391-71

150 Tablets

Tegretol© 250mg

carbamazepine
Chewable Tablets

CAUTION: Federal law prohibits dispensing without prescription.
Usual Dose: Adults 1-2 tablets

Container 2

NDC0663-5391-71

150 Tablets

Tegretol© 255mg

carbamazepine
Chewable Tablets

CAUTION: Federal law prohibits dispensing without prescription.
Usual Dose: Adults 1-2 tablets

Using the labels above, circle the correct answers below.

1- Tegretol tid but no more than 765mg in 24-hr

Container 1 or **Container 2**

2- Tegretol q4h no more than 1.55g – How many mg are given in a single day?

a. 1050 c.1550
b.1350 d.1530

Container 1 or **Container 2**

3- Give 0.3g stat of Tegretol

Container 1 or **Container 2**

Notes/Calculations

Scored Tablet: A Tablet that is scored (There is an indention or cut in the tablet) so that it may be split evenly in half.

It is important that you only cut tablets that are scored otherwise the tablet will not be evenly split and as a result you will not be accurate in the amount of the medication you are giving the patient.

Consider the chart below in reference to scored tablets and fill in the "amount to give".

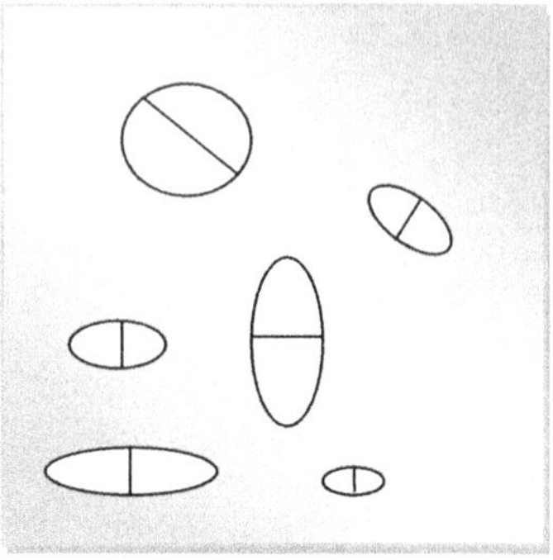

Scored Tablets

Scored Tablet Calculations

Doctor's Orders	*Tablet Concentration (Scored)*	*Amount to Give*
0.5mg	1mg per tab	0.5 tab (1/2 the tablet)
125mg	25mg per tab	
2.5g	500mg per tab	
3g	250mg per tab	
150mg	150mg per tab	
0.5g	500mg per tab	
0.5g	1g per tab	
250mcg	50mcg per tab	
30mg	60mg per tab	
0.1g	250mg per tab	
0.15mg	0.3mg per tab	
450mcg	225mcg per tab	
150mg	300mg per tab	
1g	250mg per tab	

Notes/Calculations

Calculating the amount of mL to give a patient is similar to the 7 step process for the Dimensional Analysis that we discussed on page 9 of this book. We will now just add another step that will allow us to analyze liquid medications.

Steps	**Process**
1	Identify the desired units for the answer
2	Identify your 'On-hand" units
3	Identify the needed conversion factors →
4	Determine the correct structure for the problem
5	Estimate the answer
6	Perform the necessary mathematics
7	Evaluate the answer and compare to your estimated answer

<u>**Step 3a**</u>: determine the medication ratio – (5mg per 5mL OR 100mg per 5mL).

<u>**Step 3b**</u>: order or dose to be given.

Example:

Ordered: Oral syrup 8mg stat for a patient with stomach pain.

$$\frac{mL}{Dose} \qquad \frac{5mL}{5\cancel{mg}} \Bigg| \frac{8\cancel{mg}}{1\,Dose} = \frac{40}{5} = \boxed{8mL}$$

NDC0613-5361-74

175mL

Drug XX©

Oral Syrup

5mg / 5mL

CAUTION: Federal law prohibits dispensing without prescription.

Usual Dose: Adults 5-10 mL

Notes/Calculations

Example:

1- <u>Ordered:</u> Zofran Oral Solution 7mg PO qhs for allergies

NDC0663-5391-71
75mL
Zofran©
Ondansetron hydrochloride
Oral Solution
3mg / 5mL
CAUTION: Federal law prohibits dispensing without prescription.
Usual Dose: Adults 5-10 mL

$$\frac{mL}{Dose}$$

2- <u>Ordered:</u> Tylenol Oral Solution 70mg PO qhs for allergies

NDC0663-5391-71
325mg per 10.5 mL
Tylenol©
Acetaminophen
Elixir, USP
Oral Solution
325mg
CAUTION: Federal law prohibits dispensing without prescription.
Usual Dose: Adults 10-15mL

$$\frac{mL}{Dose}$$

3- <u>Ordered:</u> Robitussin Oral Solution 80mg for a Cough

NDC0663-5391-71
100mg per 5 mL
Robitussin©
Cough & Cold
4FL oz. (118 mL)
Oral Solution
30mL
CAUTION: Federal law prohibits dispensing without prescription.
Usual Dose: Adults 10-15mL

$$\frac{mL}{Dose}$$

Notes/Calculations

Dose to be given	Concentration	Conversion	More Less Same	Amount to give
0.35g	**350mg per mL**	**0.35g = 350mg**	**Same**	**1mL**
825mg	**0.5g per mL**	**0.5g = 500mg**	**More**	**1.65mL**
2500mcg	**1.5mg per mL**			
3000mcg	**2.5mg per mL**			
0.15g	**425mg per mL**			
200mg	**50mg per mL**			
0.1g	**200mg per mL**			
100mg	**500mg per mL**			
650mg	**150mg per mL**			
0.4g	**200mcg per mL**			
525mg	**10mg per mL**			
0.5g	**650mg per mL**			

Practice Example

Dose to be Given:	**825mg**
Concentration:	**0.5g per mL**
Conversion:	**0.5g = 500mg & 1g = 1,000mg**

$$\frac{\text{mL}}{\text{Dose}} \rightarrow \frac{1\text{mL}}{0.5\text{g}} \bigg| \frac{1\text{g}}{1000\text{mg}} \bigg| \frac{825\text{mg}}{\text{Dose}} = \frac{825}{500} = \boxed{1.65\text{mL}}$$

Notes/Calculations

Not all medication is pre-prepared and ready for administration from the medicine vials. You may be required to mix the medication with another solution (another drug or sterile water).
To effectively dilute or mix the medication you need to understand the meaning and application of percent, fraction, and ratio.

Term	Meaning	Examples
Percentage	**"Out of 100" or "per 100"**	**20% - 50% - 76%**
Fraction	**Part of a whole number**	**½, ¾, ¼**
Ratio	**Compares values**	**1:1, 1:4, 1:2**

Doctor orders:
250mL of Drug X at 50%
You would prepare 125mL of Drug X and 125mL of water. It could also be written as 1:1 ratio or ½ strength of Drug X.

Doctor orders:
Epsom Salt @ 1:4 bid
1:4 = 1 part Epsom Salt and 4 parts Water.
1 + 4 = 5 Total parts
Fraction of 1/5
percentage of 20%

Fill in the Chart below:

Doctors Order	Percentage	Fraction	Ratio
50% of Drug X	**50%**	½	**1:1**
20% of Drug X			
1:2 of Drug X			
1/5 of Drug X			
1:1 of Drug X			

Notes/Calculations

Hypodermic	Beneath the skin
Insulin Syringe	Smallest syringe - 0.3 to 1mL
Intradermal (ID)	Shots between the dermis and the epidermis of the skin (TB Shot)
Intramuscular (IM)	Shots into the muscle (Flu shots)
Intravenous (IV)	Injection into the vein (Fluids or other medications)
Needle Gauge	The thickness or diameter of the needle (The higher the gauge, the smaller the needle is)
Parenteral Medication	Injectable medication (Use of a needle)
Subcutaneous	Injection of medication below the dermis and the epidermis layers of the skin. (insulin shots)

Layers of the skin and other tissues

Skin layer	Shot Type
Epidermis	**Hypodermic**
Dermis	**ID**
Subcutaneous	**Subcut**
Muscle	**IM**

Notes/Calculations

The equipment used will depend on the type of medication to be given, the route it is to be given, and the amount that is to be given. There are medicine cups, syringes (needleless and needle), and droppers.

In the chart below is some general information about some different syringes that are commonly used.

Syringes

Calibration: 0.5ml per line **Purpose:** Feeding the patient via tube **Route:** Tube **Type:** Needleless	60mL Syringe
10mL Syringe	**Calibration:** 0.25 per line **Purpose:** administration of medication or saline flush **Route:** IV Push & Oral **Type:** Needleless
Calibration: 0.2ml per line **Purpose:** Injection medication and/or oral **Route:** IM & IV Push & Oral **Type:** Needle or Needleless	5mL Syringe
3mL Syringe	**Calibration:** 0.1 per line **Purpose:** Injection medication and/or oral **Route:** IM & IV Push & Oral **Type:** Needle or Needleless
Calibration: 0.01 per line **Purpose:** Inject of insulin medication **Route:** Subcutaneous **Type:** Needle	1mL Syringe

Calibrations of Syringes:

1- Locate the 1mL marking on the syringe
2- Count the number of lines below the 1mL line

$$\textbf{1mL} = \frac{\text{1mL}}{\text{100 calibrations}} = \text{0.01mL per calibration}$$

$$\textbf{3mL} = \frac{\text{1mL}}{\text{10 calibrations}} = \text{0.1mL per calibration}$$

$$\textbf{5mL} = \frac{\text{1mL}}{\text{5 calibrations}} = \text{0.2mL per calibration}$$

*Knowing the calibrations is extremely important because you need to measure the medication to the nearest 10th of a mL.

Notes/Calculations

Size	*Color ID*	*Gage*
●	Olive	14
●	Amber	15
●	Grey	16
●	Green	18
●	Pink	20
●	Purple	21
●	Blue	22
●	Orange	23
●	Red	25
●	Clear	27
●	Lavender	30
●	Yellow	32

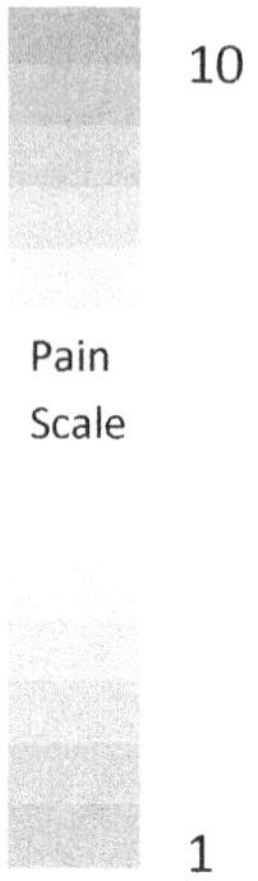

Type	Length
IM	1-2 inches
Subcutaneous	3/8 – 5/8 of an inch
ID	3/8-1/2 of an inch

There are 4 main IM injection sites.

Thigh (*vastus lateralis muscle)*	**Top of upper arm** (*deltoid muscle)*
Hip (*ventrogluteal or gluteus medius muscle)*	**Buttocks** (*dorsogluteal muscle)*

Notes/Calculations

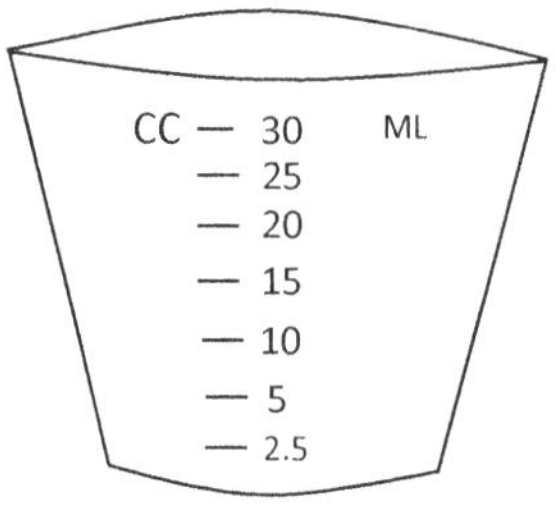 	**Calibration:** 2.5 – 5 mL per line **Purpose:** administration of liquid medication **Route:** Oral **Type:** Cup

You will often need to give the patient a specified medication dose that can't be measured in a cup alone, either the dose is above or below the markings of the cup. If that is the case, use the steps below to administer the correct amount of medication.

<u>Steps to administer oral liquid medication in a cup & syringe</u>

Prescription Pad

Give the patient 14.5 mL of oral cough syrup daily for three days.

X *Dr. Ray Bradley*

1- Prepare 10mL in the cup
2- Use a 5mL syringe to draw 4.5mL
3- Add the 4.5mL to the cup
4- Administer 14.5mL of medication to the patient

Using the medication cup shown above, fill in the graph below.

Dose to be given	Amount in cup	Amount in syringe	Syringe size 3mL or 5mL
14.5mL	**10mL**	**4.5mL**	**3mL**
14.4mL			
20.1mL			
2.5mL			
16.8mL			
22.9mL			
26.3mL			

Notes/Calculations

NDC06654-1254-42 75mL ***DRUG X*** Oral Solution **3mg / 5mL**	**NDC**06654-1254-42 75mL ***DRUG Y*** Oral Solution **4mg / 10mL**

I don't know about you but I hate shots... Hate them! So, if I need a shot of two different medications and it can be combined into one syringe then you can bet your bottom dollar I will have them combined. *Not all medication can be mixed.* Ask your supervisor if you are unsure.

Two medications One Syringe (Steps)

Prescription Pad

Drug A 1.5mg
and
Drug Y 0.5mg

X Dr. Ray Bradley

1- Work out calculations for *Drug X*
2- Draw appropriate amount of mL into syringe
3- Work out calculations for *Drug Y*
4- Draw appropriate amount of mL into syringe
5- Administer medication in one shot to the patient

Drug X	**Drug Y**	**Administer**
$\frac{mL}{Dose} = \frac{5mL}{3mg} \Big\vert \frac{1.5mg}{Dose} = \frac{7.5}{3} = \frac{2.5mL}{Dose}$	$\frac{mL}{Dose} = \frac{10mL}{4mg} \Big\vert \frac{0.5mg}{Dose} = \frac{5}{4} = \frac{1.25\ mL}{Dose}$	2.5mL + 1.25mL **3.75mL**

Notes/Calculations

Using the two different drugs shown on page 69, fill in the graph below.

Drug X	Drug Y	Amount in syringe	Syringe Size 3mL or 5mL
1.5mg	0.5mg	3.75mL	5mL
3mg	-	5mL	5mL
-	1.5mg	3.91mL	-
0mg	-	0.75mL	3mL
1.8mg	0.4mg	-	3mL
1.2mg	-	4mL	5mL
-	0.6mg	5mL	-

Show your work

Notes/Calculations

Continuous IV Infusion:	Just as it says, an IV that flows continuously until ordered otherwise.
Drop Factor: (DF)	The amount or number of drops per mL delivered through an IV.
Electronic Infusion Device: (EID)	A machine that delivers IV fluids and or medication at a set rate. $EID = \frac{mL}{Hour}$
Flow Rate:	The rate at which medication or fluids are being delivered through the IV.
Gravity Infusion Device:	A device that uses gravity to infuse the fluids. (Drop Factor, Macrodrip, Microdrip)
Infusion Line: (Primary)	The main IV line that is connected to the patient.
Infusion Line: (Secondary)	Plastic tubing that connects to the main IV line. This connection port allows additional medication or fluids to be administered to the patient without the use of additional injections.
***IV piggy back*:** (IVPB)	50-100mL medication bag infused through a secondary infusion line.
IV Push:	Delivering additional medication through a secondary IV line. All the medication is delivered at once but could be over a 1-2 minutes.
Macrodrip: (Gravity Infusion)	IV drops that are 10-20 drops per mL.
Microdrip: (Gravity Infusion)	IV drops that are 60 drops per mL.
Osmolarity:	The concentration of a solution- similar to ratio, fractions and percentage.
TKO	"To Keep Open"
KVO	"Keep Vein Open"

Notes/Calculations

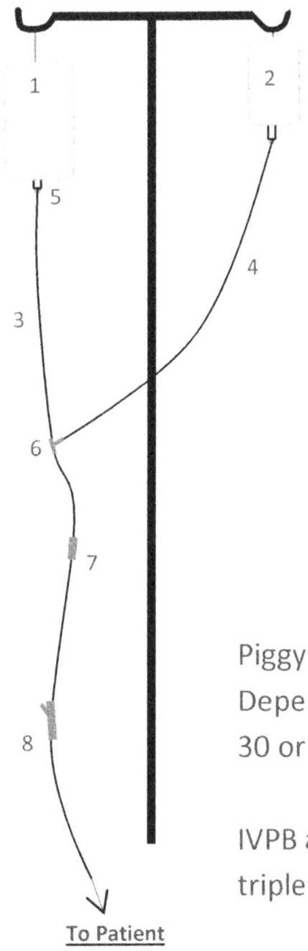

Number	Name
1	Primary Bag
2	Secondary Bag
3	Primary Line
4	Piggyback Line
5	Micro/Macrodrip chamber
6	Piggyback Y Port
7	Clamp
8	Secondary Port

Piggy Back solutions come pre-prepared in volumes of 50mL and 100mL. Depending upon the order, you will infuse the secondary bag over 20, 30 or 60 min.

IVPB are infused based on the Flow Rate; we can simply double or triple the mL per hour

Order	(Triple) 20 min	(Double) 30 min	60 min
100mL IVPB over__min	300mL per Hour	200mL per hour	100mL per hour
50mL IVPB over__min			
20mL IVPB over__min			
60mL IVPB over__min			
30mL IVPB over__min			

Notes/Calculations

There are three things to know when calculating IV therapy.

Flow Rate → Volume → Time

*In order to find the Flow Rate you will need to know the amount of fluids (Volume) to be administered and the duration (Time) of infusion.

$$\text{Flow Rate} = \frac{\text{Volume}}{\text{Time}}$$

Mathematically the Flow Rate is written out as either $\frac{\text{mL}}{\text{Hr}}$ (EID) OR $\frac{\text{Drops}}{\text{Min}}$ (Gravity).

Doctor's order: Give patient 1L of D5W every 8 hours.

Prescription Pad

Give patient 1L of D5W every 8Hrs.

X *Dr. Ray Bradley*

- No mention of drops so we know we are using an EID machine.

-We know that 1L is the same as 1,000mL so we can use the mL per hour setup.

- We DO NOT know the Flow Rate to set the EID at.

$$\frac{\text{mL}}{\text{Hr}} = \frac{1000\text{mL}}{8\text{ hr}} = \boxed{125\text{ mL per Hour}}$$

Doctor's order: Set EID at 120 mL per hour with a 500mL D5 bag.

Prescription Pad

Set EID at 120 mL per hour with a 500mL D5 bag.

X *Dr. Ray Bradley*

-We know the Flow Rate and Volume.

-We DO NOT know the Duration.

$$\text{Time} = \frac{1\text{hr}}{125\text{mL}} \times \frac{500\text{mL}}{1} = \boxed{\textbf{4 Hours}}$$

Notes/Calculations

Order	Flow Rate	Volume	Duration
Infuse 1000mL NS over 8 hrs	125mL per Hour	1000mL	8 Hours
Infuse 500mL NS over 5 hrs			
Infuse 120 D5W over 8 hours			
1L of NS q8h			
500mL of D5 at 40mL per hour			
Infuse 5000mL NS over 15 hrs			
1L of NS q4h			
1000mL of NS q8h			
1000mL of D5 at 40mL per hour			
325mL of half strength NS q6h			
Infuse 500mL NS over 8 hrs			

Show your work

Notes/Calculations

Whether you are using a EID device or gravity to infuse the medication or liquids, you will still need to know the Flow Rate, Volume and Time. However, rather than the Flow Rate being expressed in mL per hour ($\frac{\text{mL}}{\text{Hr}}$). It will be expressed as drops per min ($\frac{\text{Drops}}{\text{Min}}$).

There are two different types of drip chamber sizes. Microdrop and Macrodrop.

Macrodrop

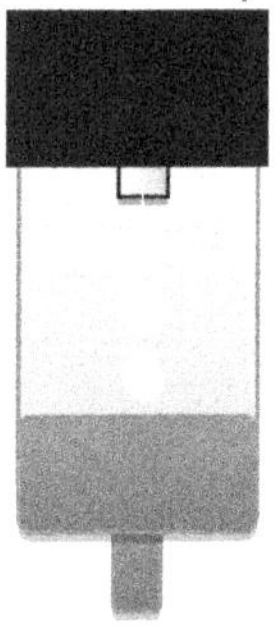

$\frac{\text{10 - 20 drops}}{\text{mL}}$

Microdrop

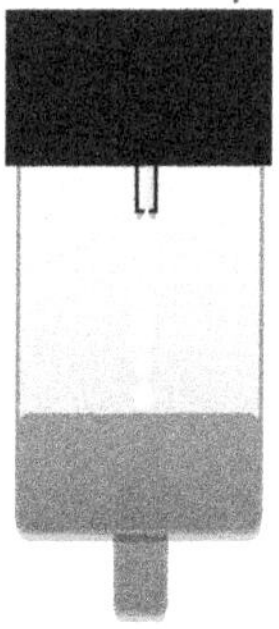

$\frac{\text{60 drops}}{\text{mL}}$

<u>**Doctor's Order**</u>:

Infuse IV 500mL over 5 hours on a gravity device. Set the Drop Factor at 15.

Flow Rate	Volume	Duration	DF
100mL per Hour	500mL	5 Hours	15

$$\frac{\text{Volume}}{\text{Time}} \left\{ \frac{\text{Drop}}{\text{min}} \right\} \qquad \frac{100\text{mL}}{1\text{hr}} \times \frac{1\text{hr}}{60\text{min}} \times \frac{15\text{Drops}}{1\text{mL}} = \boxed{\text{25 Drops per min}}$$

Flow — Time (Conversion Factor) — DF

Notes/Calculations

Using what you know about Drop Factors, fill in the chart below.

Doctors Order	Flow Rate	Volume	Duration	DF	Drops Per Min
Infuse 500mL over 5hours. DF = 15	100mL per Hour	500mL	5 Hours	15	25
Infuse 1000mL NS over 5hrs DF = 10					
Infuse 120mL D5W over 8 hours DF = 15					
1L of NS q8h DF = 15					
500mL of D5 at 40mL per hour DF = 20					
Infuse 5000mL NS over 15hrs DF = 60					

Show your work

Notes/Calculations

Often medication is administered orally or IV based on the weight of the patient. Because we use Kg to describe the weight of the patient you will need to be able to convert pounds to kg before you calculate the amount of medication or fluids to administer.

Example:

A patient weighs 100 lbs, how many kg does he weigh?

$$\frac{100\text{ lbs}}{} \left| \frac{1\text{Kg}}{2.2\text{ lbs}} \right. = 45.5\text{Kg} \qquad \frac{45.5\text{Kg}}{} \left| \frac{2.2\text{ lbs}}{1\text{Kg}} \right. = 100\text{ lbs}$$

Some medications are based on what is known as <u>Safe Dose Range</u> (SDR). The Drug will state a range of mg that are safe for a patient based on their weight.

SDR Example:

<u>Order</u>: Drug Y, 0.25g tid (250mg)

<u>SDR</u>: 10-20mg/kg/day in 2-3 divided doses

$$\frac{145\text{ lbs}}{} \left| \frac{1\text{Kg}}{2.2\text{ lbs}} \right. = 66\text{Kg}$$

Your Patient

Age: 30

Sex: Male

Height: 5'6"

Weight: 145 lbs.

Range:

Low: 10 x 66 = 660mg/day in 2-3 divided doses

High: 20 x 66 = 1320mg/day in 2-3 divided doses

250mg tid(3) = **<u>750mg/day</u>**

Now we ask ourselves if our 250mg given 3 times a day (750) falls within the SDR of 660mg – 1,320mg. Yes it does. So we are good to give it to the patient.

If the medication falls below or above the SDR then you need to consult with the prescriber and make Notes/Calculations according to what the doctor says.

Notes/Calculations

Fill in the chart below. Refer back to page 85 if needed.

Order	SDR	Patient Weight (lbs)	Patient Weight (kg)	SDR	Dose Ordered	Give?
Drug Y, 0.25g tid	10-20mg/kg/day in 2-3 divided doses	145	66	**Low:** 10x66=660mg/day in 2-3 divided doses **High:** 20x66=1320mg/day in 2-3 divided doses	**750mg**	**Yes**
Drug Y, 200mg bid	5-10mg/kg/day in 2-3 divided doses	200				
Drug Y, 0.5g tid	25-50mg/kg/day in 2-3 divided doses		50			
Drug Y, 0.55g	25-50mg/kg/day in 2-3 divided doses	105				
Drug Y, 0.5mg q6h	1-2mg/kg/day in 2-3 divided doses		14			
Drug Y, 100mg q4h	8-12mg/kg/day in 4-6 divided doses		63.5			
Drug Y, 0.25g tid	10-20mg/kg/day in 2-3 divided doses	165				
Drug Y, 0.35mg tid	5-10mg/kg/day in 2-3 divided doses	109				
Drug Y, 0.35g tid	10-20mg/kg/day in 2-3 divided doses	125				

Notes/Calculations

Medication that is administered based on weight is not limited to SDR only. Depending on your selected field of nursing, you could be administering IV infused medication on a daily bases. Review the sample problem below then do the follow up problems. Take Notes/Calculations as to how many Conversion Factors are used.

Ordered: Drug A IV Infusion 0.5mcg/kg/min/day
On Hand: Drug A 250mg/200mL.
Patient weight: 110 lbs

$$\frac{110\text{ lbs}}{} \bigg| \frac{1\text{kg}}{2.2\text{ lbs}} = 50\text{kg}$$

$$\frac{\text{mL}}{\text{hr}} = \frac{200\text{mL}}{250\text{mg}} \bigg| \frac{1\text{mg}}{1000\text{mcg}} \bigg| \frac{0.5\text{mcg}}{\text{kg} * \text{min}} \bigg| \frac{50\text{kg}}{1} \bigg| \frac{60\text{min}}{1\text{hr}} = 1.2\text{mL per hour}$$

Work the Problems out below:

Ordered: Drug A IV Infusion 0.5mcg/kg/min/day **On Hand**: Drug A 250mg/250mL. **Patient weight**: 100 lbs	
Ordered: Drug A IV Infusion 1.5mcg/kg/min/day **On Hand**: Drug A 250mg/100mL. **Patient weight**: 110 lbs	
Ordered: Drug A IV Infusion 3.5mcg/kg/min/day **On Hand**: Drug A 250mg/150mL. **Patient weight**: 150 lbs	

Notes/Calculations

Let's say it is 0800 and your shift ends at 1300. You have been asked to infuse 1000mL of NS q10h. You know that your shift ends in 5 hours. Not only do you need to correctly calculate the infusion rate (mL per hour) but at what time the 1000mL will be completely done infusing so you can report this to the nurse who follows your shift.

Catch Up Time

Now let's say that you make your rounds and return to the patient's room to check in the EID device and the infusion rate and discover that there is now 750mL remaining in the bag and the time is 1100. Ask yourself these questions.

1- Is this the correct amount of mL to have at this time to end at 1800 hours?
2- What is the difference, + or -?
3- At what Infusion Rate do I need to set it at to ensure that the NS will be done infusioning at 1800?

Target Volume	Volume remaining	Difference + or -	New Infusion Rate
700mL	**750mL**	**50+ mL**	**107mL per Hour**
Time Passed X Infusion Rate Volume Spent Volume Spent - Total Volume Target Volume 3 Hours X 100 mL/hr 300 mL 300 mL - 1,000 mL 700 mL	Look at the IV Bag 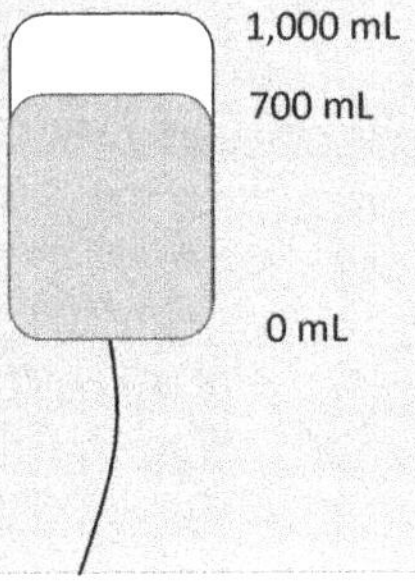	Volume Remaining - Target Volume Volume Difference 750 mL - 700 mL 50+ mL	Volume Remaining / Time Remaining = New Rate 750 mL / 7 Hours = 107 mL per hour

Notes/Calculations

Pg. 7

1. milli 2. Kilogram
3. kilo 4. milli
5. kilogram 6. L
7. One tenth of a liter
8. One Millionth of a gram

9. mL 10. mcg
11. g 12. mg
13. L 14. Kg

Pg. 15

1. 12in/1Ft
2. 1km/0.6 mile
3. 16oz/1 lbs

Pg. 17

1. 5mL 2. 3tsp
3. 90mL 4. 100,000mcg
5. 2.5cm 6. 100cm
7. 700mg 8. 0.1g
9. 400cm 10. 4m
11. 30.48cm 12. 2.5cm

Pg 19

1. 36inches
2. 4000ml/ gal
3. 91.44cm
4. 30.48cm

Pg. 21

1. 96tsp
2. 350,000mcg
3. 0.00027g
4. 0.274L
5. 165lb
6. 7.5mm

Pg. 23

1. 27.432m
2. 25.4mm
3. 4 cups
4. 2340 inches
5. 6.8Kg
6. 210 seconds

Pg. 25

1. 1g
2. 3g
3. 0.4g
4. 0.35g
5. 2000mg
6. 800mg
7. 145mg
8. 50mg

Pg. 27

1. 1800mg
2. 800mg
3. 3600mg
4. 6mg

Pg. 29

1. 8.61g
2. 0.91g
3. 0.025g
4. 1.801g

Pg. 31

1. 0.0028g
2. 0.02g
3. 0.005g
4. 0.0235g

Pg.33

1. 350mL
2. 68tbs
3. 1.75oz
4. 1500mL

Pg.45

1. A
2. A
3. 03, 03, 09,12, 15, 18, 21, 00
4. Now
5. Now and then every 6 hours

Pg. 49

1. Either
2. D, Container 2
3. Container 1

Pg 51

1. 0.5 2. 5
3. 5 4. 6
5. 1 6. 1
7. 2 8. 5
9. 0.5 10. 4
11. 0.5 12. 2
13. 0.5 14. 4

Pg 55

1. 11.67mL
2. 2.26mL
3. 4mL

Pg.57

1. 1.5, 1500mcg
2. 2500mg/ml, 1.2
3. .425g, 0.35
4. 4mL
5. 0.2, 0.5
6. 0.2 mL
7. 4.33mL
8. 0.0002g, 2000ml
9. 52.5
10. 0.65, 0.77

Pg. 59

1. 20%, 1/5, 1:4
2. 33%, 1/3, 1:2
3. 20%, 1/5, 1:4
4. 50%, ½, 1:1

Pg. 67 1. 10 in cup, 4.4 in syringe, 5mL 2. 20, .1, 3mL 3. 2.5,cup or syringe 4. 15, 1.8, 3mL 5. 20, 2.9, 3mL 6. 25, 1.3, 3mL **Pg 75** 1. 0 2. 0.1mg, 5mL 3. 0.3mg 4. 1mL 5. 0.8mg, 4mL 6. 2.1mg , 5mL **Pg 75** 1. 150, 100, 50 2. 60, 40, 20 3. 180, 120, 60 4. 90, 60, 30 **Pg 79** 1. 100mL/hr, 500mL, 5hr 2. 15mL/hr, 120mL, 8hr 3. 125mL/hr, 1000mL, 8hr 4. 40mL/hr, 500mL, 12.5hr 5. 250mL/hr, 5000mL, 20hr 6. 250mL/hr, 1000mL, 4hr 7. 125mL/hr, 1000mL, 8hr 8. 40mL/hr, 1000mL, 25hr 9. 54mL/hr, 325mL, 6hr 10. 62.5mL/hr, 500mL, 8hr	**Pg 83** 1. 200mL/hr, 1000mL, 5hr, 10, 33.3 2. 15mL/hr, 120mL, 8hr, 15, 3.75 3. 125mL/hr, 1000mL, 8hr, 15, 3.75, 31.25 4. 40mL/hr, 500mL, 12.5hr, 20, 13.33 5. 250mL/hr, 5000mL, 15hr, 60, 250 **Pg 87** 1. 91, Low=5*91=455mg, High = 10*91=910mg, 450mg, No 2. 110, Low=25*50=1,250mg, High = 50*50=2,500mg, 1.5g, Yes 3. 48, Low=25*48=1,200mg, High = 50*48=2,400mg, 0.55mg, No 4. 31, Low=1*14=14mg, High = 2*14=28mg, 2g, No 5. 140, Low=8*63.5=508mg, High = 12*63.5=762mg, 600g, Yes 6. 75, Low=10*75=750mg, High = 20*75=1,500mg, 0.75g, Yes 7. 49, Low=5*49=245mg, High = 10*49=490mg, 1.05mg, No 8. 57, Low=10*14=570mg, High = 20*57=1,140mg, 1.05g, Yes **Pg. 89** 1. 1.36mL/hr 2. 1.8mL/hr 3. 8.59mL/hr

Made in the USA
Monee, IL
05 November 2026

67375694R00057